The Burnout Recovery Kit

Practical help for dealing with the epidemic of our time

John Ardent

ISBN-13: 978-1-98107-053-4

DEDICATION

For my parents, who watched over me during my darkest hours; and
Stephen, my wonderful cousin whom stress and anxiety took down a tragic
road.

CONTENTS

DISCLAIMER

The content of this book is designed to provide helpful information and encouragement on the subjects discussed. This book is not meant to be used, nor should it be used, to diagnose or treat any medical condition. For diagnosis or treatment of any medical problem, consult your own physician. The publisher and author are not responsible for any specific health or allergy needs that may require medical supervision and are not liable for any damages or negative consequences from any treatment, action, application or preparation, to any person reading or following the information in this book. References are provided for informational purposes only and do not constitute endorsement of any websites or other sources. This book is not intended as a substitute for the medical advice of physicians. The reader should regularly consult a physician in matters relating to his/her health and particularly with respect to any symptoms that may require diagnosis or medical attention.

CHAPTER 1 – WHY I WROTE THIS BOOK

INTRODUCTION AND ENCOURAGEMENT

In March 2004, I suffered a life-changing nervous breakdown as a result of burnout from work-related stress and exhaustion. It marked the beginning of my darkest hour, yet also the start of a lifelong journey of increased self-awareness and personal liberation.

At the time, I began searching bookshops for answers to describe what on earth was happening to me. Unhelpfully, my doctor consulted the basic instruments of his profession and informed me I was absolutely fine. As you will soon discover, that was most definitely not the case. Several collapses, seizures and trips to the hospital later, and I finally got an inkling from medical professionals that what I was going through was surprisingly common. In fact, it is no exaggeration to describe burnout as 'the epidemic of our time.' In the fast-paced, information-overloaded modern western workplace, that is most definitely an accurate description.

Countless scholarly volumes have been written on the topic, and I could recommend many of them myself. This little book is intended neither to compete with nor replace them, rather as a complimentary aid. As I waded through various texts during my illness - trying to put together some sort of natural recovery plan - I wished I could find a work that addressed me where I was presently at. A book that would hold my hand in a very lonely place, and shine a light on ways out of a seemingly hopeless pit of despair.

Eventually my doctor attempted to prescribe a course of sleeping pills and anti-depressants, but I refused to take them. The hospital consultant stated that he expected me to be off work for at least a year, even with the aid of medication. I returned to 'light duties' in the workplace after five months with no chemical assistance whatsoever, through a mixture of determination, discipline, the love and support of family, and several common techniques described throughout this text.

I should stress that while I was quickly working a full week again, this was not in my previous intensive position as a software developer (a role I never returned to). However, both local medical professionals and the Human Resources department at my workplace were fairly well astounded. So much so, that in the years and re-thought career that followed, I was periodically called upon to get alongside others evidencing a bit of a 'wobble' in regard to their own wellbeing.

Right from the very start I wish to make it clear that refusing medication was a personal decision I made because it seemed right for me at the time. Countless people continue to benefit from taking prescriptions during burnout, and many lives have undoubtedly been saved as a result. There were moments during the heaviest hours of my illness when very insistent thoughts of suicide came to the fore. Thankfully I was able to resist, but it could easily have gone the other way while my brain chemistry was in such a mess. If you are experiencing such thoughts, PLEASE speak to family, friends, medical professionals or anyone else you trust. In such a situation, anti-depressants may be just the lifeline you need to find a safe equilibrium. Under different circumstances or without the presence of my wonderful family, I may also have made a choice in favour of the meds. The key word in the title of this book is 'RECOVERY.' I want to help you get to a place of wellness. There are no prizes for refusing drugs, and I'm not a better person of bigger man because I just happened to do so.

If you haven't already studied the 'Disclaimer' at the start of this book, I encourage you to please go ahead and review it. I am not a medical professional nor qualified practitioner in any of the techniques described hereafter. All I am is a regular guy who researched a lot of alternative or complimentary ways to claw his way out of a very dark place, and used them to restore some semblance of normality to his life. This book describes how I did it. Maybe some of that will help you too?

One kind soul once suggested a course of 'me' should be

available on prescription from their doctor. Naturally I cannot be with you in person during your hour of need, and that was the inspiration behind this text. A work many people have encouraged me to write for a number of years.

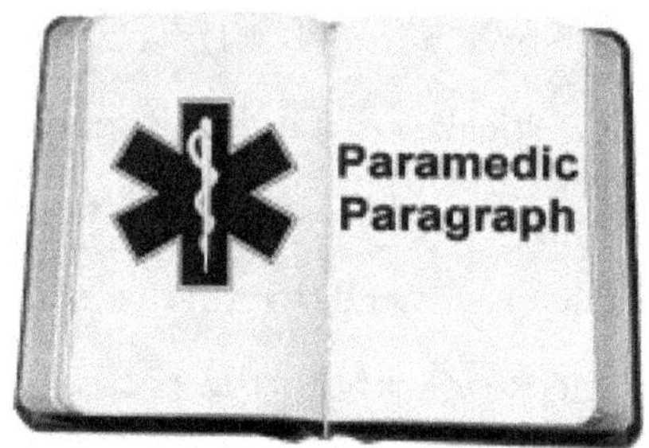

Chapters 3 – 7 feature these sections known as 'Paramedic Paragraphs' at the very start.

When I suffered burnout, scanning through copious amounts of text to find helpful exercises in books was just another barrier to my recovery, at a time I could barely face such a seemingly simple task.

Thus I have elected to place variations of the assorted practical exercises that helped me, at the very start of a chapter. They are written in italicized text with a helpful symbol alongside to draw your eye to them.

These are taken from well-known natural techniques used the world over, including Cognitive Behaviour Therapy (CBT), Neuro-Linguistic Programming (NLP), and others.

If you want to read more about that particular technique and how it fits into my story, you will find details in the rest of the corresponding chapter. But if all you need at that moment is an exercise to help, it should make your life that much easier.

The subtitle to this chapter was *'Introduction and encouragement.'* With the former fairly well covered, let's look at the latter via the medium of several key facets related to burnout I have found to be personally true. Ones that many discussions with others who have undertaken a similar journey most definitely reinforce:

Your life will NEVER be the same again.

At first that sounds particularly scary, or as if recovery is impossible. Not a bit of it! For the most part your life will never be the same again, but in a very good and helpful way. Strange as it may sound, burnout is something of a gift. Right now you might feel like returning it if you possibly could! When I was off sick, a kind lady at work sent me a 'Get Well' card. Inside she wrote a simple phrase that I clung onto: *'Don't worry, the clouds will part and the sun will come out again.'* And you know what? She was absolutely right. If you take nothing away from here other than that simple phrase, you are already onto a winner.

Your life will never be the same, because you are about to become a whole lot more self-aware in relation to your personal physiology than you have ever been before. You will instinctively know when a situation is healthy and/or works for you, and in some cases even find yourself able to detect that in others (certainly my experience). That said, this doesn't make us infallible from bad decisions or the ability to ignore that inner voice. Once you've taken a trip down 'Burnout Lane,' you are more susceptible to paying another visit. I can't stress enough how important it is to listen to the new voice of your body. Though in the modern workplace, it is not always easy to have things our way. Most likely (through no deliberate fault of your own) you got where you are through not hearing/heeding your own internal warnings, until your world came crashing down. Some wholesale changes may lie ahead.

Stress happens.

Sounds pretty obvious, but there it is. The stress response goes back to the 'fight or flight' process that is part of our innate survival mechanism when faced with threatening situations. However, today this mechanism gets activated by situations one wouldn't necessarily associate with 'survival' as such. Our systems are flooded with Adrenaline, Cortisol and Norepinephrine, all of which are designed to help us fight a threatening encounter, or run away successfully where it would be foolish to do so. Having our bodies continuously pumped full of those chemicals can have negative, long-term health consequences. Continuously heavy workplace stress is one such trigger. The bad news is that stress can happen anywhere. When I first fell ill, I was desperate to avoid all stress. While that is a sensible desire when initially recovering from burnout, as a long term strategy it is sadly unrealistic. Any facet of life can include some types of stress from time to time. A little stress is even beneficial in helping us achieve our goals. The important thing is to learn how to deal with that stress, both physically and mentally. There were weeks in my post-recovery revised career where things periodically became very stressful. However, through the application of everything I learned on the way to wellness, I found that I mostly knew how to cope and get through. In time and with a little practise, you will also develop new skills and resilience to help survive similar moments. It is only where such situations are continuously going from bad to worse, that more drastic, permanent life changes might need consideration.

You are neither weak nor a failure.

Burnout seems crazy and just doesn't make any sense. In a world where people are expected to be tough and independent, it can make you feel like a big, fat failure. However, burnout typically happens to talented, hard-working people who are really good at and committed to their jobs. One thing you may encounter if/when you return to your previous workplace, is a common prejudice against anyone with an 'invisible injury.' You haven't got an arm in a sling to wave around, and everything from comments about malingering through patronising put-downs to full-on accusations of retardation are sadly possible. I enjoyed all of those curious pleasures. The other 'chestnut' is the subtle (and sometimes not so subtle) suggestion that you just aren't cut out for the workplace. I would argue that the modern workplace is rarely cut out for people, but more on that at the end of the book. One amusing observation I made over the years, is that many individuals who deliver such slights are professional slackers. People who got where they are by riding the wave of (or even taking full credit for) the hard graft and innovation of others, don't typically suffer from burnout. They talk a good game, but talking is about all they do. Sooner or later many are 'found out,' and move onto another job where they can pull the same trick until they are discovered again. Caring about the job not being done right and carrying the extra workload caused by these deadbeats, may have even been a contributing factor to your illness in the first place. Thankfully on my own team we had no such people as a causative factor, but I certainly encountered them during my onward workplace journey. When there is no praise flying around to appropriate, these losers definitely don't want the spotlight shining anywhere near their own indolent incompetence. Diverting attention to somebody with a perceived weakness – such as a colleague who has previously suffered burnout – seems to be a fairly common ploy. In a variation on an old cliché: Burnout isn't a sign of weakness; it just means you've been strong too long.

If you haven't experienced burnout, you CANNOT appreciate it.

This sounds a little harsh at first. Many people who love and care about you are hopefully doing everything they can to help. Medical professionals well-schooled in all facets of burnout/nervous breakdowns etc. may have lots of great advice and suggestions for you. But, the fact remains that unless they have personally and individually been through it themselves, they CANNOT appreciate it. You may already have a sense of what a lonely place you are in, and how nobody around you really understands. That's because they most likely do not. It's one big reason I wrote this book in the first place: to be a companion. The semi-good news is that you are part of a growing 'club,' with more solidarity about than you might presently realise. One of these days you will probably meet another burnout sufferer. When you do, ask them whether or not the statement in bold type above is true. I'm sure you won't have to, because you already know it is…

So, how did my own journey start? In the next chapter we'll take a look.

CHAPTER 2 – WHAT'S HAPPENING TO ME?

MY DESCENT INTO DARKNESS

"John?! John?! Whoa, steady mate, it's Dave. You're alright, I've got you." The disembodied words of reassurance echoed through a black void. My body shook in a violent fit. Though my eyes were open, they had rolled back in my head. All I could see was darkness, and at that moment I had absolutely no idea who or where I was. As consciousness slowly returned, I became aware of firm but kind hands securely resting on my upper arms to try and ease the spasms. The harsh feel of a rough, training school classroom carpet informed my senses that I was now sat on the floor. Gradually, light and focus returned. All around me, nine other peers from various parts of the organisation sat in their course seats, looking down with faces that evidenced a mixture of emotions.

"You made a funny noise in your throat, then fell back in the chair with your head jammed underneath an electrical conduit on the wall," the gentle words of my manual handling trainer spoke again as he released my

arms. *"We helped you down onto the floor as you started to fit."*

The classroom door opened. An admin assistant entered to notify Dave that an ambulance was on its way.

I had barely been in the class forty minutes or so. It was a half-day course on revised manual handling techniques, which many staff from across our 6,500 strong employer would be required to attend. The trainer was an acquaintance who normally worked a couple of buildings away from my own office. He barely got through an introduction to spinal components and how they can be damaged, when this first episode in my life-changing journey struck.

I had really been looking forward to the course. It meant a morning out of the office, away from a job I was reasonably good at but absolutely hated. I was a senior software developer, previously given an award for my work around eight months prior. Earlier that week, a colleague found me with my head in my hands. When he asked what was wrong, I simply replied, *"I just can't face another day of looking at that screen."* Writing and de-bugging thousands of lines of code from Monday to Friday was taking its toll. Our unit were victims of our own success, and subject to constant (and frequently very impolite) demands for new custom software delivered to impossible timescales. Everyone wanted a piece of our work, and issuing threats seemed a good way to jump the two year backlog of job requests. On the way to work the day of my episode, I had resolved to speak with my boss that afternoon and ask for at least a six month secondment to another unit. The penny had finally dropped inside that if I didn't get out, something bad was going to happen in regard to my health. Unfortunately I had left it too long, and was now beyond the point of no return.

Two paramedics entered the classroom and conducted a series of checks, including blood pressure and sugar levels. I didn't know at the time, but the 'finger prick' test was soon to become all too familiar. After being placed on oxygen, I was taken down in a wheelchair to the waiting ambulance. Dave escorted us, asking if there was anyone I would like him to call. I apologised profusely for having disturbed his course so thoroughly. He told me not to worry about it. A colleague called Martin said he would collect my belongings and drive over to accompany me at the hospital Accident and Emergency Unit. It was a kind and much-appreciated gesture. One I have never forgotten.

Whether from the effects of the oxygen, the jostling ride, or possibly a mixture of the two, I had the distinct pleasure of vomiting in the back of the ambulance. A few days later I would get a ride to another hospital, in a different ambulance with another crew. It was at this time I fully realised what incredible people paramedics are, and how under-appreciated they can often be in our society. Their reassurance in those difficult and confusing moments, was more than words can tell or thoughts guess.

Martin found me at A&E. He sat trying to cheer me up with a joke or two, and further described what happened in class. The attending physician did another set of examinations, instructing me to get some rest and see my doctor for a follow-on check-up. After making sure I wasn't intending to drive, he released me.

When Martin and I returned to the office, I managed to phone my brother-in-law for a ride home. It was at this time that I felt particularly lucky that 'home' was still my parents' house.

Like many of my peers I had left school, gone out to work, and done all the usual things a conscientious young man my age did to get on. However, following cutbacks at a previous employer some years before, I took voluntary redundancy to fund a college course in the United States. This morphed into several years working in different countries on a penniless, voluntary basis, giving something back to those in need. Eventually my sister and her husband bought a home, and I began thinking about the future.

I took a temporary IT training job on a one year contract, which I loved. Since there was no chance of making it permanent, I looked at other posts in the same organisation. When the chance to sit an exam to see if I could make the cut as a software developer was put to me, I took one look at the money and permanent prospects and thought it was worth a shot.

A couple of years on, I observed the housing market heating up, cleared a car loan and started shopping for a home. After our employers stiffed the team on a pay rise we had been promised, I lost the little house that additional money would have secured. Looking back, it probably did me a favour. I don't envy anyone who lives alone with a massive mortgage hanging over their heads, particularly if they then get a walloping dose of burnout. If that describes you, dear reader, rest assured you have both my heartfelt sympathy and utmost admiration.

Sure enough the housing market went positively into orbit. Even couples with two good incomes found it hard to buy, and I ended up burning the candle both ends to try and play catch-up with a runaway train. It was never going to work. Today that same tiny house is three times what I would have struggled to pay for it, but the staff in my old unit earn pretty much the same wage we did then. Utter madness…

As difficult as it sometimes felt after living around the world and knowing one's independence, I was never more grateful for my wonderful childhood home and family than during that period of illness and total exhaustion.

My doctor was about as much use as the proverbial chocolate teapot. He grudgingly agreed that I should come in for a blood test with the nurse, but said there didn't appear to be anything wrong with me.

Ever since the classroom collapse, I had been very shaky on my feet and not entirely coherent. Putting words together into a sentence suddenly began to feel like a gargantuan task, and it appeared to be getting worse rather than better. My father insisted on driving me to the nurse and coming in for the blood test. I was in no state to protest. I suspect even the thought of his dazed son crossing a road with such a foggy brain, was cause for concern.

The nurse's room was very hot. My internal temperature gauge appeared to have become ultra-sensitive. There was some suggestion of possible thyroid issues, which the blood test would reveal.

I had never been squeamish about blood, and would ordinarily watch it extracted from my arm into a syringe without blinking. The nurse asked me to sit in a chair as she began the procedure. I have no idea at which point I had another blackout and seizure, but the description from my father bore many similarities to those of the classroom incident. Apparently I made a funny noise in my throat, my head lolled back, then I started to fit violently and unconsciously ripped the needle out of my arm. Once again everything went black. I could hear my father's voice trying to calm me down, as he and the nurse attempted to hold me steady in the chair. When my sight returned, the look of concern on the woman's face was both touching and worrying at the same time. She commented that ripping the needle out of my arm must have been extremely painful. To be honest, I was feeling increasingly numb all over and disconnected from the world around me. Vaguely aware of a sharp pain from the needle wound, it seemed the least of my worries at that particular moment.

Dad drove me home, and explained what had happened to my mother. I suddenly found that my limbs had begun to lose sensation. Walking across the room to the toilet took an age, as I wobbled and held onto furniture for support, unable to properly feel my own legs. Speaking had grown increasingly difficult, and if I was asked a simple question such as: *Would you like a cup of tea?* I found it a mammoth task to try and decide whether I did or not. If I began speaking and got interrupted mid-flow (suddenly everyone around me appeared to talk at a hundred miles an hour, without listening), it was so confusing and stressful I couldn't even continue. So it was that I said as little as possible, or gave up at the slightest hint of anything that felt mildly like an interrogation.

Saturday evening, the numbness began spreading from my legs upwards. It felt like death invading and paralysing my body, and was extremely worrying. Later that night when it reached the base of my neck and I found it nearly impossible to move, my parents decided not to mess around and phoned for an ambulance.

Sure enough: more tests and 'finger pricks,' plus another ride with an equally fabulous paramedic crew who did their utmost to provide comfort and humour. If they'd just driven around the block in circles talking like they were, I think it would have done more for me than many hours spent in A&E during the busy Saturday night/Sunday morning shift.

My folks followed along in a car, sitting up and watching their son connected to monitors throughout the night.

It is at this point I should mention the genuine care of a

lovely Ghanaian nurse serving in A&E that Sunday morning. Throughout this little book, you will read testimony of how stress and anxiety can have dramatic and sometimes debilitating effects on human physiology. One simple, everyday component we're probably all familiar with, is the effect of nerves on the bladder. Like everything else during burnout, this can be frequently amplified in certain situations.

A seemingly indifferent orderly handed me a disposable bedpan when I asked to use the loo. Even with curtains drawn around the casualty bed, my system was too wired to release the pent-up stream. Thus I found myself in significant discomfort with growing pressure on my bladder, but no environment conducive to relieving it. When I asked the orderly again if I could use the loo, he informed me it was the bedpan or nothing. In a confused and agitated state, this was not what I needed to hear.

A few minutes later, a Ghanaian nurse (my family discovered her origin after thanking the woman later) emerged with a warm smile. After hearing of my quandary, she considered the pathetic-looking figure on the bed with thoughtful eyes.

"Okay. I'm not really supposed to, but I can take you to the toilet and wait outside while you go."

She was absolutely lovely. Breaking policy and rules with a simple act of kindness that meant so much to me, I felt the need to include it here, fourteen years later. Already I had begun to realise that the tiniest things (good or bad) appeared to have greatly exaggerated impacts on my entire being, with whatever was happening to me.

More 'finger pricks' followed, along with the extraction of blood for an in-hospital test. Thankfully I didn't blackout and have a seizure this time, not even when the bloodied victims of a nasty car crash were wheeled past on trolleys.

Morning wore on and my family left as I was transferred to the Clinical Decision Unit while staff waited for various test results. That evening I was placed in another bed, alongside a window full of holes. If you are familiar with British weather during early March, it was like trying to rest next to an open car window on a motorway drive during frost. I attempted to stuff paper tissues into as many of the cracks as I could to stem the blast, wondering how on earth anyone could manage a night there. And that from someone who has slept in some pretty rough places during his travels in the third world!

Eventually a specialist arrived on his rounds with some student/junior doctors. He took one look at me, read my chart and nodded knowingly. It was about the most reassuring look I have ever received.

"Can you try walking from the bed to the wall?" he asked.

Some of the feeling had returned slightly, so I managed to wobble across the ward a few paces. The specialist's next words to me (especially considering he knew nothing about my occupation) were utterly astounding and really rather telling.

"Do you work in I.T?"

I nodded.

"Are you a programmer?"

I nodded again, unsure of where this was going or if the man was perhaps psychic in some bizarrely medical manner.

He turned to his crowd of followers. *"Classic case of nervous exhaustion."*

Looking at me again, he continued. *"What's happening, is your body is shutting down and stopping you, before you stop, PERMANENTLY. You've been overdoing it. Very common situation among I.T. workers. Humans aren't meant to work at the same speed as computers. I see they were considering a CT scan tomorrow. Well, I think what you really need is to go home for a period of absolute rest that you won't get in hospital. I will arrange an appointment for you to see me in a couple of weeks. If we need further tests at that time, so be it. But, I've seen this kind of thing many times before."*

Clearly he wasn't kidding. It came as some relief to know I wouldn't be spending a night next to that dreadful, draughty window. How an elderly person would have coped, I have no idea.

When I eventually met the specialist again as an outpatient a few weeks later, he informed me that I needed a complete change. I was told in no uncertain terms that if I reached the stage where this happened to me again, he would rather not be held responsible. The destination next time being the morgue rather than A&E, or at the very least my fatal demise from a stress-induced heart attack before the age of forty, if I survived another collapse.

First though, I was looking forward to getting home and finally catching up on some much needed sleep.

As it happens, that would be the one thing which proved largely impossible for the next three weeks.

We'll look at that next, and how to break the vicious circle of sleeplessness and subsequent further exhaustion when your nervous system is utterly frazzled.

CHAPTER 3 - TO SLEEP, PERCHANCE TO DREAM

BREAKING THE VICIOUS CIRCLE OF SLEEPLESSNESS

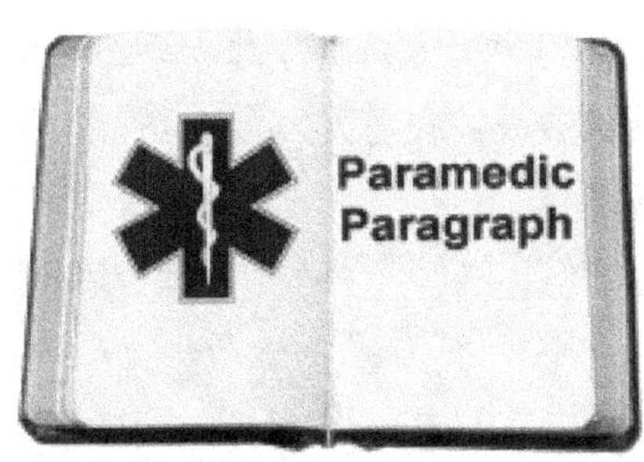

Progressive Muscular Relaxation (PMR).

This technique helps to relax your mind and body by tensing then relaxing various muscle groups throughout your frame, in sequence. The basic premise is that by manually tensing muscles for a few seconds (5 – 10 is typical) then feeling them relax, you also naturally let go of associated anxiety and mental tension.

I highly recommend using this in concert with 'Circular/Diaphragmatic Breathing' (see start of Chapter 6) as a dynamite combination for a good night's rest.

I have put those techniques in a separate chapter, as they are a wonderful tool you can use anywhere during a panic attack (for example: while out shopping), without arousing undue attention.

Remember: *You don't need to read the whole of Chapter 6 to pick up that technique, so by all means take a look at the 'Paramedic Paragraph' there first and come back to this, if you find that helpful. The basic key is to slow and control your breathing as part of this powerful process. As long as you can currently take long, even breaths and release them, that will do just fine for now.*

Choose a place/time where you won't be interrupted for at least ten to twenty minutes. Ideally, if you can lie down on your back and stretch out comfortably, that is a bonus. I have however done this successfully while sat up in a chair on nights I just couldn't lie down, so you don't have to be in bed.

Believe it or not this even works on the floor. However, if you are planning to get to sleep as part of the process, you might want to consider another location.

Although this can also be performed at any time for anxiety and tension relief (rather than sleep), it is advisable to be in a situation without distractions such as TV or nearby external conversation.

If you have a special piece of music that helps to relax you, that is a possible addition. However, make sure you can safely leave it to finish without having to get up and turn equipment off afterwards. The point of this exercise when used for sleep purposes, is to relax your body down into undisturbed, restful unconsciousness.

If you use music, I would also recommend avoiding tracks that evoke strong mental imagery (even positive imagery), for the following reason:

The most important facet of this exercise is maintaining a consistent mental focus on your body. By visualizing each muscle tense and relax as you physically do it, you will find the positive effects amplified considerably. Anything that interrupts that mind/body connection, can lessen the benefits.

You are going to tense, hold and release muscles starting at your toes and gradually working upwards towards the face. This will help identify tension, which can creep up on you and be surprisingly difficult to distinguish. Unconsciously walking around with muscles tensed all the time is not a great way to live, as I'm sure you can appreciate.

The important thing is not to get disheartened if PMR doesn't produce immediate results. This is normal, and it took me a week or so before I could really notice any benefits.

Just consider the exercises as an investment in your long-term recovery, and keep doing them. Once the effects kick-in, they are well worth the tenacity and discipline required, I can assure you.

Some proponents of this method use long, drawn out scripts. During burnout I found these not particularly helpful, as you can't memorize or assimilate a lot of new information. Typically I ended up worrying more about if I'd missed something, rather than focusing on the exercise in question.

Therefore, I'll keep this deliberately simple and allow your own mind to adapt the imagery as you go.

First, memorize the following instructions, so you can put the book down and do it. Let's begin.

1. *Start by breathing in slowly, holding your breath gently, and letting it out again. If you want to ensure the rhythm is even, count to five as you breathe in and hold, then five again as you slowly let the breath go. Continue to do this throughout the remainder of the exercise.*

2. *Curl and tense the muscles in your toes, then relax. Do the same with your feet and ankles. Feel and imagine the tension draining away and let them go loose and heavy.*

3. *Continue to do likewise with your calves, thighs and legs.*

4. *Next move up to your hips, buttocks and lower back, remembering to tense and release each in turn, letting go and imagining you are like a ragdoll.*

5. *Still breathing slowly, tighten and release your stomach. As you reach your chest to do the same, notice the gentle rise and fall with the action of inhaling and exhaling.*

6. *Hands, arms, shoulders and neck come next. Take your time with each. Don't rush.*

7. *Finally we arrive at the face. Tense your forehead into a crease and let go. Tense your jaw and do the same. Screw up your eyes, then feel the relaxation as you slowly release them.*

8. *Now shift focus to encompass your whole body. Tense everything at once, then feel it go loose and heavy, sinking down into whatever you are laying/sitting on. It's not unusual to have a sensation of weightlessness at this stage. Enjoy it! Take a few additional long, slow, even breaths. If you are planning to get up (for example doing this momentarily during the day), I suggest counting backwards from five and allowing your mind to gradually notice the surrounding environment you are in. This makes*

it a bit less of a shock to the senses. Otherwise, allow yourself to continue relaxing, and (hopefully) get some much needed sleep.

When I first started doing this exercise, smart phones and tablet computing hadn't been invented, and the Internet contained a lot less material. These days you can find free, online audio recordings of complex relaxation scripts (typically on common video sites) that can be played through headphones while doing this, should you wish. This adds value to such scripts and requires zero memorisation, so if that works for you then great!

By deliberately stripping PMR down to its basic elements above, I have given you an easy-to-remember method that can be employed anywhere with zero equipment. This was what I did in 2004, because the copious pages of printed scripts were too large and intimidating to remember during my episode. Did it work? Well, we'll get to that in a moment. First a bit of background for the exercise above.

PMR was invented by American physician, Dr. Edmund Jacobson, whose work is largely responsible for the word 'relax' attaining its current, modern English meaning in common parlance. He wrote a number of books on the topic, including 'Progressive

Relaxation' in 1929 which included detailed procedures for the removal of muscular tension that he first presented at Harvard University in 1908. The underlying idea is that muscle tension is commonly a psychological response to stress and anxiety, translated into a bodily manifestation. By reversing the process (i.e. relaxing tensed muscles) we can release the tension and help reduce or even stop the impact of further stress/anxiety on our system.

PMR is commonly used to treat insomnia, as either a complimentary or alternative method to pharmacological interventions. 'Racing Thoughts' are a frequent side-effect of burnout, but also other illnesses that interrupt sleep patterns. This technique has been used to provide some relief to cancer patients also, where pain-induced insomnia is an issue. The increased blood flow and supply of oxygen the technique produces, can even lessen pain and muscle spasms.

As well as 'Progressive Muscular Relaxation' – sometimes called 'Progressive Muscle Relaxation'- Jacobson also invented 'Biofeedback.' He died on 7th January 1983, aged 94.

When I arrived home from hospital, the thought of finally getting some rest and that the 'problem' with me had now been identified, provided some reassurance. It was when I climbed into bed that the cruelty of this condition reared its ugly head. One minute I was hot and sweaty, the next cold and shivering. Covers on, covers off, up and down like a yo-yo as I tried to regulate an unstable temperature. Try as I might, it seemed impossible to quieten the mind. This wasn't a new experience, as my career in software development made it impossible to switch off. There were always routines, coding, ideas, solutions, insane work schedules, pressures, etc. running on an endless, chaotic loop through my frazzled brain. This played no small part in the nervous drain which led to that first collapse, when my personal resources to 'cope' were finally overcome.

Now, as my head hit the pillow and I began slipping into unconsciousness, a surge like electricity would fire through my nervous system and immediately snap my body awake again. Much later I discovered the term 'Hypnagogic Jerk.' While this sounds like some sort of insult, it is also the technical term for what I experienced. Typically the experience is shortened to 'Hypnic Jerks' or labelled 'Sleep Starts.' These involuntary muscle twitches are a bit like being startled from behind when a joker sneaks up on you. Hot flushes and sweats followed, along with a frequent sensation of falling. There I was back at square one, trying to drift off to sleep again. As soon as I did? You guessed it: another 'Hypnic Jerk.'

I had been up all night and the following day in hospital, and was already suffering from nervous exhaustion anyway. Now, the one thing I needed more than anything to get well, seemed to be the one thing I couldn't do: SLEEP.

A week later I had managed next to no sleep and was at my

wits end. At night I sat up in a chair, hoping to drop off because lying in bed was just so frustrating. My energy and emotional state hit rock bottom.

The Sunday after that return from hospital, my sister and brother-in-law came round for a visit. I was sat in a chair as usual, dazed and quiet, wondering what on earth was happening or if I would ever get well. As my sister approached to say goodbye, I clung onto her from where I sat. Moments later I began sobbing my heart out. It was a shock to a sibling who hadn't seen me cry since we were young children. Tears in her own eyes at the state of me, she said *"We'll get you well yet, don't worry."*

My brother-in-law placed a firm and reassuring hand on my shoulder. *"You get some rest and keep your chin up."*

The quivering wreck before him was a startling contrast to the joking, bubbly, confident man who had helped fix-up their first house, and regaled crowds with witty anecdotes as 'Best Man' at his wedding the year before.

What little sleep I managed, was barely restful. The 'Hypnic Jerks' were an almost constant companion, made worse by worrying about them. It's the classic 'Catch-22' like TRYING to fall asleep. The harder you try, the more difficult it becomes.

I attempted all manner of things to alleviate the problem: warm baths, scented candles, relaxing music etc. One night I finally drifted off into a peaceful slumber that felt great, only to be awoken an hour later by our drunk neighbour crashing around next door and shouting at his wife. Afterwards, I wasn't able to sleep again. Like I really needed another challenge…

With no real improvement in sight (and still waiting for the follow-up specialist appointment I mentioned in the last chapter), I decided to go and see my local doctor again. He needed to sign me off work for another couple of weeks anyway. The surgery was very warm as usual. Now, I began to notice that due to my experiences there, I had built a mental association with passing-out and such environments. I'll get more into that when we look at 'Stress Triggers' in the next chapter.

As I sat in the waiting room, the nurse who had taken my blood saw me and hurried over. Her face appeared grave with concern.

"Are you alright?"

It transpired she had never had a situation like that seizure during my blood test. Her inquiry was heartfelt.

My doctor on the other hand, was his usual, useless self. From bronchitis to burnout, whenever I paid the man a visit, we always had to have a big fight until he finally discovered that there WAS in fact something wrong with me each time. Do people really just go to visit their local surgery for fun/a chat, I wonder? Doesn't seem very likely. I wasn't equipped for a big battle on that particular day. Having no useful advice or knowledge relating to my condition to offer, he grudgingly prescribed some sleeping pills and anti-depressants to help me rest. At first I collected them, but eventually decided that it wasn't the right path. I'm terrible at taking pills anyway, but something inside just said *"No."* Not listening to my inner voice was one reason I had reached such a low place, so this time I was 'all ears.' My choice, my consequences, my responsibility. The drugs might have helped, but I was determined to find a natural way out of that dark pit.

A couple of days later, my folks were off on a trip to a nearby country town. Though I looked a sight - pale, wan and spaced-out, shuffling around - they asked if I'd like to come along for a spot of fresh air. While there, I found a lovely old bookshop and began rifling through the medical/psychology section for anything with possible/practical answers. That was how I happened upon PMR, and marked the start of learning a variety of techniques to help on the path to victory. As I have previously mentioned, the 'relaxation scripts' I found were unwieldy to someone struggling with even basic dialogue and attention due to their illness. However, I managed to summarise the gist, understood the purpose, and distilled them into something I could start using. A definite case of necessity being the mother of invention, I believe. Basically, the result looked very similar to the eight simple steps I listed at the start of this chapter.

At first it felt nice to release the tension, but there was no dramatic improvement in my insomnia from attempting PMR. I kept at it. About a week or so later, I woke up realising I had managed about four hours of continuous, undisturbed rest. It was only a little 'fuel in the tank,' but the sense of achievement alone boosted the experience and lifted the emotional clouds considerably.

There were certainly days when it seemed as if I had gone backwards. This proved a common theme on the way to recovery, and if/when it happens to you, don't beat yourself up about it. 'Three steps forward, two steps back,' is still one step forward. Hang onto little nuggets like that. They are an absolute life-saver.

Gradually, inch by inch, it felt as though I had managed to start climbing from rock bottom to the faint glimmer of light far above. On the way I would discover that activities and situations I had once taken for granted, now began to produce a dramatic and very real negative physical and emotional response when I encountered them. That's what we'll take a look at next.

CHAPTER 4 - RE-PROGRAMMING YOUR AUTOPILOT

CHANGING HOW YOU REACT TO STRESS TRIGGERS

Graded Exposure.

This technique is a way to confront stress triggers that sometimes develop from neuroses burnout gives birth to.

Once-ordinary situations and activities can be subconsciously associated with the cause of our stress/anxiety, leading to powerfully negative emotional and physical reactions when those things are encountered.

This is especially awkward when the situation or activity is a fairly normal and necessary one, resulting in a pattern of avoidance. In an attempt to protect ourselves, we can seriously limit our life options in some pretty unhelpful ways, unless a solution can be found to address those reactions.

Fortunately, by gradually easing into such situations and activities in a measured manner with specific achievement milestones, it is absolutely possible to conquer our fears. By so doing, we can break the negative mental associations and their corresponding automatic physiological responses.

There's no magic exercise or anything special to remember here, just a simple process as follows:

1. *Identify your stress triggers.*
2. *Detail SMART objectives on the way to conquering them.*
3. *Break each objective down into a series of smaller steps.*
4. *Once the objectives are achieved, create new ones that take you further towards conquering the fear completely (if you haven't already done so).*
5. *Repeat steps 2 – 4 until the trigger no longer fires when you encounter it.*

The beauty with this is that you get to chart your own progress, which has the additional benefit of raising your mood and clearly illustrating that you are on the path to recovery.

If you are unfamiliar with SMART objectives, they are a way to ensure a milestone has certain key qualities, as follows:

***S** – Specific (Can the goal be accurately described, rather than just being a woolly ideal?)*

***M** – Measurable (Can it be measured to see if we have achieved it?)*

***A** – Achievable (Is it realistic? Few things are more discouraging than failing to achieve something because the bar was set too high in the first place)*

***R** – Relevant (Does the objective have appropriate bearing on our ultimate goal?)*

__T__ – Timed (Having an objective that is set in the 'never never' is of little use. Sometimes deadlines are helpful).

Let me give you an example of how I put this in to practise, to help you draft your own.

One of my neuroses revolved around using computers, for fairly obvious (if slightly daft) reasons. In classic burnout 'all or nothing' stress thinking, I found myself having panic attacks and turning into a quivering, sweating mass of jelly, curled up in the foetal position if I even entered a room with a computer close by. And that was with the machine switched off!

So, my ultimate goal was to be able to use a computer normally again (for whatever purpose), even if I didn't go back to programming work. This had nothing to do with returning to the job which caused my problems in the first place, just conquering one of the negative spin-off side effects from the illness. Many aspects of life involved using a computer then, and even more-so now. Thus, not freaking out while in the presence of such machines was a fairly important state to achieve.

To be able to operate a computer normally, I would obviously have to first be in a room with one.

Thus my initial SMART objective read something like:

'By next Thursday, I will be able to sit in a room with a computer switched off for ten minutes, while still remaining calm and composed.'

The small steps along the way were broken down into shorter durations of the overall objective (i.e. Day 1 — spend two minutes in the room. Day 2 — spend four minutes in the room etc.)

Some days you will have a hiccup and go backwards. Don't worry, that's normal. Just do the last step you managed for a couple more days before trying again. Alternatively, your steps might be a little large. Break the next step into two smaller ones and see how you go. Tick off every successful mini milestone reached, celebrate, give yourself a pat on the back, and look at the paper of ticks regularly.

Once I achieved my ten minutes, I wrote a new SMART objective for ten minutes with the computer switched on etc. Then twenty minutes. Then ten minutes touching the computer (perhaps turning it on then off). Gradually it grew into opening a simple document then shutting down, and so on.

Whatever your stress triggers, there are ways to confront them in a manageable and uplifting fashion.

My two others were driving alone and warm environments, mainly due to fear of passing out and having another seizure. I created goals, SMART objectives and baby steps for each of those.

Eventually I conquered the lot.

Despite sounding like some dreadful, corporate management exercise; this stuff really does work on the journey to burnout recovery!

I walked into the bedroom and my eyes fell on the switched-off computer in the corner. Suddenly, my whole world turned upside down without warning. Sweating profusely, shaking all over, I sank to the floor in the corner with my back to the wall. Waves of fear and adrenaline coursed through my body. Tears rolled uncontrollably down my cheeks. I rocked back and forth, hugging my aching chest. What on EARTH was going on?!

Welcome to the wonderful world of stress triggers! If burnout itself doesn't seem to make any sense, these little babies are the most ridiculous, embarrassing, and confusing of all. Everyday situations and activities you once took for granted, just became panic-inducing phobias without asking your permission first.

Here was a man who worked on the most complex software in a variety of programming languages as 'Senior Technical Analyst,' used computers creatively for writing and video production in his spare time, and now couldn't even be in the same room as one without turning into a trembling puddle of nerves. It was an unpleasant revelation, to say the least.

When I next went to get another work sign-off slip from my doctor, I ended up having to stand outside in the cold and have someone come and get me once the appointment was due. Waiting in the warm surgery environment induced the same set of physiological responses as my experience with the computer. By this time, the thought of getting behind the wheel of a car alone did pretty much the same. Despite a long drive to work each day, this was not specifically associated with the cause of my exhaustion. However, since I had twice collapsed into a fit without warning, the fear of that happening on the road clearly became an issue and joined the other new phobias. In such a low state, I wasn't overly concerned about losing my own life. But, the prospect of injuring or killing another person due to my illness was simply unthinkable.

A few days later, I received an appointment to visit the Medical Officer on-site at our employer's headquarters. The MO was an external, qualified doctor who spent a certain number of hours a week working to assess and aid staff for the organisation. This covered the whole gamut of injuries, both visible and invisible, and enabled them to provide appropriate care for staff while meeting legal and organisational HR employment requirements. During the period of my recovery, I actually got to meet three different MOs. The first quit over alleged pressure to sign unfit staff back to work, the second went off with (wait for it) WORK STRESS, and the third was thankfully still there after I fully returned to operational duties in a new job role.

The MOs had seen people in my condition countless times before, though commented that I had suffered at the absolute sharp-end of just how bad burnout can get. It was such a relief to get some positive advice and guidance from medical professionals. The impartiality of their not being organisational employees, also provided genuine reassurance that somebody was on my side. People without an agenda to shoe-horn me back into that dreadful and wholly unsuitable old job, ASAP.

By this time I had visited the hospital specialist as an outpatient, and been advised to ditch my career in software development. I honestly didn't need to be told that; it was patently obvious I would never go back. However, hearing it from the lips of an expert who read me like a book before I even said anything to him while in hospital, provided another shot in the arm of confidence.

It was now late spring/early summer, and the MO gave me a brilliant recommendation that bears repeating:

"Get outdoors in the sunlight as much as possible. The light level inside is typically between 100 – 1,000 lux. Outdoors on a clear day, it is 10,000 lux. Vitamin D absorbed from being in such an environment can act as a significant mood enhancer, and help with rest, relaxation and recovery."

She was absolutely right. It is worth adding a caveat here to take appropriate precautions against UV rays etc. if you are planning on doing the same. I didn't sunbathe at all, or even stay outside in direct sunlight for long. But, even sitting outdoors under a shade on a warm day with good light, provided a marked improvement in subsequent sleep and general well-being.

After this sage little turn of phrase, she then set me a project. At the time I didn't fully understand why, but it later made perfect sense. I informed her that I had been going for a walk with my father each morning at a nearby nature reserve full of birds, just to get some fresh air. Her eyes lit up.

"Excellent. I would like you to get a bird book, and try keeping a log of how many of each type you identify on your daily walk. Next time you visit, we will have a look at the results."

There are three very common tools for combatting psychological symptoms, which fall under the general heading of 'Distractions.' By the time stress triggers are formed, the physical reaction in your body seems absolutely automatic. Yet, the simple fact is that there was nothing a computer could do – in and of itself – to produce the kind of manifestations I experienced. The symptoms felt real, the physical exhaustion causing them was definitely real, but the cause was purely a psychological association. Think of it a bit like typing the wrong address into a web browser. Your system has started firing off a link to a blog on horror fiction, when it should be visiting a site about chocolate recipes. The key is intercepting the 'browser' and correcting the address, before your brain hits 'SEND.'

Along with the reduction in symptoms provided by graded exposure techniques listed at the start of this chapter, the three ways of doing this I mentioned are as follows:

1. Physical Activity
2. Mental Activity
3. Refocusing Activity

Constant worrying thoughts can feed and help defeat your

recovery from burnout, as well as giving strength and validity to stress triggers. Distracting a busy mind with something completely different and ideally pleasurable, is a great way to get some respite.

'Physical Activity' is a mood enhancer, can use up surplus adrenaline generated by worry, and aids the healthy functioning of the body. This doesn't necessarily have to be a sport or strenuous task. Going for a gentle walk in pleasant surroundings works just as well. While in the throes of burnout, you will most likely find yourself intensely aware of when you've had enough physical exercise, and when you definitely would benefit from more. Even another 'turn around the block' can be helpful.

'Mental Activity' is the process of engaging your mind in something completely un-related to the source of your problems. Reading a nice story, reciting an old, favourite poem memorized in childhood, engaging in a relaxing hobby requiring the recall of specific steps and attention, remembering happy occasions and situations while attempting to paint all the details very vividly in your mind; all these things short-circuit the brain on its way to visiting the wrong 'website.'

'Refocusing Activity' relates to a popular and in-vogue term of the last decade or so: 'Mindfulness.' The pace of modern life, full of transient, cheap, rushed situations is a huge contributor to the stress epidemic sweeping the west. Mindfulness is all about paying very close attention to our surroundings and what we are currently doing.

When was the last time you really listened to identify all the various sounds around you? How about the feel of a certain texture or fabric against your body? When did you last slowly eat a meal in silence, fully focussing on the sensation of the food in your mouth, the aroma emanating from your plate, the subtle mixture of tastes in your mouth with every bite? How about walking down the street and looking up to observe (and really notice) all the details of the buildings above the shops in your town?

When you focus intently on something, not only can the experience be truly rewarding and generate increased happiness and appreciation for all that is in your life, but you won't be ruminating on other worries. It's simply impossible to do so, when properly paying attention to something else.

As you can probably now see, the project given to me by the MO ticked pretty much all three of these distraction boxes. By setting the task up as a daily exercise, I was definitely engaging in physical activity on my walk through the nature reserve. As the days grew bright and sunny, the Vitamin D boost also intensified. Spotting, attempting to identify and match observed birds against pictures in a book, then recording their numbers, proved a perfect example of mental activity. My attention was fully diverted to something completely unrelated to the source of the problem. Then, in the beauty of the surroundings I would often stop, shut my eyes, feel the warmth of the sun, the soft touch of a gentle breeze, smell the fresh air, listen to the call of the birds and rippling water etc.

This came quite instinctively without instruction, and thus I engaged in refocusing activity also.

My father kindly typed up the recorded birds from our notebook onto a spreadsheet, for printing and presentation to the MO. As I continued with my graded exposure plan in that regard, I was soon able to do this myself. Another achievement to celebrate!

Naturally this was just one example of a distraction project, issued by a savvy doctor who identified an additional opportunity in a routine I had already begun. It doesn't matter if you don't have a nature reserve nearby, or evidence no interest in bird spotting (I'm no ornithologist either), there will be SOMETHING you can do to receive a blessed pause from the unhelpful cacophony in your head.

Little by little, progress was being made.

When I received the first in a series of home visits from HR to encourage me back into the workplace, I had some important choices to make about what would happen next. It also meant that my recovery would now require the fragile shadow of my former self, to find a new type of resilience. Ultimately, a revised and more congruent identity. It wasn't a quick task, but probably the most important one I have ever undertaken. The reality is, that it never really ends. Change is the only constant in life, it seems. How we adapt to work with that change in a healthy manner, is the most paramount consideration of all.

CHAPTER 5 - AS A MAN THINKS IN HIS HEART

CREATING POSITIVE MENTAL ASSOCIATIONS

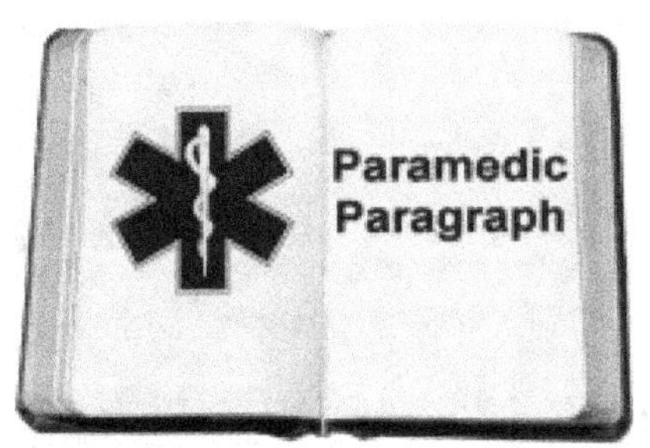

Neuro-Linguistic Programming (NLP).

NLP is often slated and supposedly debunked as a pseudoscience - inconsistent with present neurological theory - by academics who can't even agree with each other from week to week about the true nature of consciousness.

Whether it helped me for the reasons interpreted by one professor or the other, I really couldn't care less. It helped!

Here is a common technique in NLP known as 'Anchoring,' which I adapted to help myself go from barely tolerating stress triggers, to performing well in their presence. In the same way your system automatically created negative associations with certain stimuli (if you have experienced the triggers detailed in the previous chapter), we want to consciously create new associations with positive emotional, psychological and physiological responses. Effectively, we are going to train ourselves to operate with a new stimulus response pattern.

Have you ever heard someone describe a dish of tasty food, which you were then able to visualize with your mind? Did you suddenly find yourself salivating, even though there was no food in sight (or smell) of your physical senses? Congratulations, we're about to do the same thing, by associating a physical response with either an internal or external trigger of your choice.

1. *Either select one of your stress triggers, or think about a task/situation which is presently adding to your anxiety when you engage with it.*

2. *Anthropomorphise (that is to say: give form and personality to) the fear and anxiety caused by that trigger. I like to imagine the thing as a ridiculous, cartoon villain.*

3. *Now shrink the character down in size, and picture it hopping up and down like an angry ant at your feet, its voice getting squeakier the smaller it gets. Make it grey and colourless; a total, powerless loser!*

4. *Laugh heartily at the pathetic character, then stomp and squish it with your foot. You can do this with your mind if it feels uncomfortable actually stomping on nothing where you currently are.*

5. *Now imagine engaging with that trigger/task/situation and feeling how you WANT to feel about it. It might help if you can recall a situation that made you feel great, and hold onto it until you start to experience those pleasant sensations welling up inside.*

6. *Close your eyes and really amplify the image, sharpen it, make the colours richer and more vibrant, boost the sounds and let yourself feel intensely good.*

7. *Map those emotions onto the stress trigger, by imagining yourself conducting that activity while feeling how great you do now.*

8. *Finally, add an additional physical anchor by performing a gesture (I squeeze the thumb and middle finger of one hand together) right at the optimum moment of intense, feel-good energy.*

The idea behind that final step, is that it can be used to re-experience the positive feeling during any moment of stress or anxiety, not just the activity in question. If you have used graded exposure, hopefully the offending trigger is already a little less potent. By visualizing that trigger associated with feeling good, you are setting an intention of how you expect to feel while in that situation.

I would suggest repeating this step each morning before getting up. It only takes a few moments, and the day you start ACTUALLY engaging with the stress trigger with zero effort or negative effects makes it all worthwhile. If you have a wobble, use your final gesture from step 8. Once conducting this exercise becomes a habitual pattern, it is amazing to experience the hit of positive emotion by simply re-enacting this gesture.

Having 'Anchoring' as a tool in your toolbox can be useful during panic attacks, which we'll look at in the next chapter. The quick 'finger squeeze' helped me calm down and recover very rapidly on many a difficult occasion. Plus, it is a subtle action that can be used anywhere without drawing undue attention to yourself.

It came as quite a discovery when I learned that our nervous systems can't actually distinguish between a real experience and a strongly imagined one, in terms of the physiological reactions produced. This is great news. Although, you might want to keep the knowledge to yourself if trying to convince your boss that you really need a holiday. Being told to instead go and lay down on an imaginary beach for half an hour, might not be too helpful.

NLP was invented in California during the 1970's by Richard Bandler (a psychologist) and John Grinder (a linguist). Together they began modelling cognitive behavioural patterns, which formed the basis for their Neuro-Linguistic Programming methodology.

If you've understood the exercise above, you've probably already got the general idea behind the theory. Many of our responses to stimuli and situations are simply learned behaviours we automatically repeat.

After World War 2, the military discovered that many soldiers either didn't fire their weapons at all, or fired them in random directions rather than directly at enemy combatants. With the exception of a certain small number of people, it is not common human nature to be able to point a gun at another person and blow their brains out. What the armed forces required to change that behaviour, was a way of programming soldiers to automatically watch and react without thinking. Eventually this was tied in with the repetitious motion of a pop-up target, as this is similar to the way an enemy soldier might emerge from cover. When a target pops up, you point and fire. Do this enough times and it becomes an automatic response. This is a similar concept to 'Muscle Memory' in athletes and dancers, which enables them to perform complex motor tasks, without having to consciously consider the specifics.

When it comes to NLP, I like to think of it like wearing a new footpath across a patch of grass. If you go walking and find a field with a properly maintained right-of-way, the well-worn track will be obvious. This is like the well-worn paths in our neurological system, which take the same route when certain situations/stimuli are encountered, producing an identical response each time. This is one reason why I suggest repetition of the exercise at the start of this chapter. If you came to the field just mentioned, but instead took a new route across it, the grass would barely indicate your passing. The next walker may not even be aware of the track you took, and instead use the well-worn one. Keep going back to that field and walking across it in the same way however, and pretty soon a new, well-worn path will emerge. One that other walkers will also take without thinking. It's Robert Frost's classic poem, 'The Road Not Taken,' in a nutshell really.

This is what we are trying to achieve by re-programming the way our nervous systems react when encountering different stimuli. Once the new association becomes habitual (a well-worn path), pretty soon that positive result will be our automatic experience when engaging with it.

This concept of re-programming our responses, reminds me of a famous quotation from the Biblical twenty-third proverb:

'As a man thinks in his heart, so is he.'

One could easily change the gender pronoun to be neutral here of course; it applies to everyone. Our experience of what is 'real,' and how we relate to everything around us is formed largely by our habitual beliefs about ourselves, the world and others.

Winston Churchill is oft cited as the author of a similar wise saw:

'You create your own universe as you go along.'

I'm neither advocating for religious faith, nor belief in some kind of new age *'you can have it all'* teaching here (though if you partake in either, I hope they enrich you). I'm just simply indicating that what we consistently believe about life and our present situation, can have a profound impact on how we experience and habitually respond to it. When it comes to burnout: a profound impact for better or worse in relation to our recovery, the rate at which we get well, and what our subsequent life eventually looks like. Change your beliefs/automatic responses = get a different result than you would otherwise.

When the HR people came out for their first home visit, they were really rather impressed with the graded exposure goals and other methods I had worked into a loose recovery plan. Sometime later after I returned to work, one of them said, *"We didn't mind giving you a bit of extra leeway, because your genuine desire to get well and become a productive member of the organisation again was clear. In fact, we've never seen anyone quite so committed to their recovery!"*

As nice a compliment as that sounds, it wasn't all hearts and roses however. Quite clearly, they had the understandable goal of seeing this employee return to his duties in the shortest, reasonable time. It didn't matter how often I made it clear that whatever happened I wouldn't be going back to my previous programming role, the suggestion of doing so was continuously placed before me. At the time this seemed a bit scary and sinister, but taking a broader and more objective view it wasn't quite the horror show it first appeared.

If you are ordinarily a reasonably rational person and currently suffering burnout, you will no doubt be aware that you probably aren't thinking straight at this moment in time. Not a good period for making important life/career decisions, clearly. Not until you have achieved a little more equilibrium, anyway. Now imagine how you would feel if you suddenly got completely well, only to find you had quit an excellent job that you loved, based on an anxious spate of panic during your illness? I think most people would be fairly well gutted.

The hard-working folk in our HR department would push forward, then press back if I got anxious about the job suggestion, clearly testing my resilience to see if I was 'ready.'

Now, I had realised literally just before my first collapse, I absolutely had to get out of that software development position. Also, the hospital consultant pretty much told me that I needed a new career, if I liked the idea of living until middle age. It didn't matter if I had to resign from the organisation completely, or take a much lesser role doing something else, returning to the old job was non-negotiable as far as I was concerned.

Five months after that devastating classroom seizure and having taken no medication, I started work again on light duties in a temporary admin position while they monitored my recovery. All of that was achieved by liberal use of the techniques and discoveries described in this little book. The original medical prognosis was that I would be off work for a year with medication. It is no exaggeration to say that colleagues, HR and medical professionals alike were all astounded. Some years later, when I finally left that organisation for other reasons, I received the following note from a lady who knew me before the burnout, was there when I collapsed, and with whom I had several dealings in my new career later on. It read as follows:

While we didn't get much of an opportunity to work together I really enjoyed those times we did, and many's the day that seeing you being so positive helped me through. You may not realise, but your return to work was quite inspirational, for me anyway, and contributed to my 'Don't let the bastards get you down' attitude.'

I had used NLP quite extensively in getting back behind the wheel of a car, feeling how great it would be to drive anywhere I wanted without mishap (and anchoring that experience). Combining this process with 'Circular/Diaphragmatic Breathing,' 'Positive Visualisation' and 'Mental Rehearsal' techniques covered later, I was able to undertake those intimidating first few commutes fairly comfortably.

The 'HR feints' about going back to programming, made the job of dealing with my computer stress trigger that much harder. By this time I could comfortably use one for forty minutes or so, without difficulty. But, every time I made some progress, the suggestion was made about returning to the old job. This created an unhelpful mental association between using a computer normally (which I wanted to do), and being forced back into a situation that I knew was wholly unsuitable and toxic to my health. It sounds like an odd turn of phrase, but this was never 'funnier' than the day I discovered headaches from my limited computer use, were exacerbated by a need for occasional glasses to correct an astigmatism. During the eye test, my optician informed me that computer glasses would make my life a lot better. When I told HR, a delighted employee said, *"Great! Problem solved. We'll start you back as 'Senior Technical Analyst' on Monday then…"*

They weren't joking, either. I wouldn't have made it as far as lunch on day one, and I knew it.

Every time I paid another visit to the MO for my regular appointments, she looked at the case papers on her desk and shook her head at the e-mails from HR.

"Human Resources are still pressuring me about when I can sign you as being fit to return to software development. They just don't seem to get it, do they?"

So time rolled on, and I gradually grew stronger, healthier and a little more resilient. A marked improvement from the quivering lump who could barely walk, talk, or feed himself not too many months before. Eventually I think the penny finally dropped with HR that I was well enough to make a decision about the old job now, and my answer was clearly "No thanks." They had me formally resign from the position. I was classified an 'At Risk' staff member, looking for new work against a ticking clock with time running out.

Reading this, one could be forgiven for getting the impression that Human Resources at my organisation were dreadful ogres. In truth, I was so very lucky to work for the people I did. Many smaller outfits don't have anywhere near the kind of support mechanisms or staff tolerance I enjoyed. In fact, I have great affection and admiration for all the HR people who had to strike a difficult balance between my needs/requirements and those of our employer.

After trying a few quick internal IT secondments in a variety of posts, I was delighted to finally win a one year temporary contract for a new project back in the IT Training department. If the contract expired and I didn't find another job at the end, it meant I was out for good. But, this didn't matter. Finally, I was beginning a new and healthier phase in what turned out to be a very successful career. One that lasted a further eight years with the same employer.

Your own situation could well be very different from mine. Maybe you are confused about what happened, actually really like your job, and want to return to it (minus getting ill again, ideally). Your burnout might not even be related to the work you do. It is important to sit down when you feel well enough, and attempt to identify the key contributing life factors that you believe took you over the edge. As it relates to employment, there are typically three main stressors:

1. The working environment.
2. The work itself.
3. The people you work with.

Sometimes, even subtle modifications to the environment we work in can have big positive or negative influences on our mood, energy, concentration, productivity and wellbeing throughout the day. I work better in small, self-contained offices with as few people as possible. Stick me in a large, open-plan office (particularly one with bright strip lighting and a lot of noise) and I usually try to fence my desk in with books or furniture, to create some sense of privacy and personal space. I just don't work well in an environment like that. They also make me feel extra tired and very miserable by the end of the week. If I'm in a small office and also have the room to myself for a day, I will typically produce up to three times the standard workload at exemplary quality. Don't underestimate the power of your working environment to affect you.

The software development work itself clearly had a negative effect on me over time. I was reasonably well accomplished at it, but as a long term career choice nothing has ever made me so utterly miserable and depressed. Teaching IT however, filled me with energy and enthusiasm. Qualities often noted and commented on by my students. What I'm saying here, is that if you identify your actual work as being part of the problem, you don't necessarily have to go from being an accountant in London to a goat herder in the Urals before moving from drudgery to something that is a better fit. A small shift in direction that still utilises your skillset, is sometimes all you need to find relief.

I'm an introvert, so being around people for too long without respite drains me of energy. That said, I love people a great deal. I enjoy teaching and presenting to a big crowd. As long as solo recharge time is available at the end of the day, all is usually well. But if there are things which really make my working life a living hell, they are jobsworths, dishonest slackers, liars, narcissists, micro managers, and game players of all varieties. I've had some absolutely great colleagues and bosses, and some really dreadful ones too.

There is no stressor in all the world bigger than other people, and they can make or break a work situation if you don't have skin like a rhino! If you are stuck with one or more problematic colleagues - particularly rude, disrespectful, manipulative, controlling or abusive people - and can't get your employer to resolve the situation; moving on is sometimes the best thing you can do. Idiots like that are simply not worth your health. Value your skills, value your time, energy and wellbeing, and perhaps consider issuing a polite and professional ultimatum to the organisation for change. If they call your bluff, wish them well and take yourself away to a new place where you are valued instead. It's scary and occasionally disheartening if you really enjoy the work, but sometimes the only realistic choice after other avenues have been exhausted.

CHAPTER 6 – WHEN LIGHTNING STRIKES

OVERCOMING ANXIETY AND PANIC ATTACKS

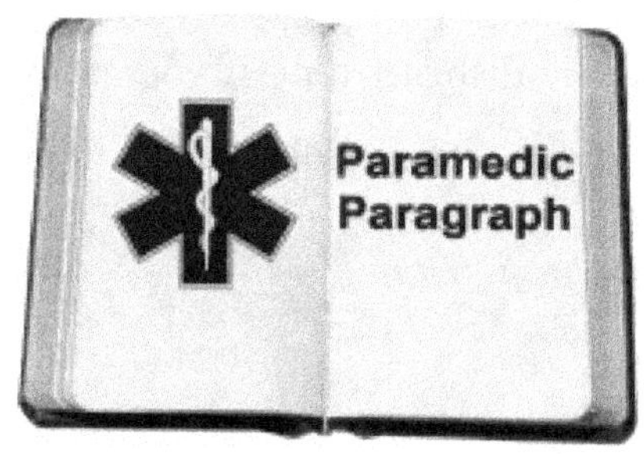

Circular and Diaphragmatic Breathing.

Ever wondered how wind instrument players, glassblowers and metallurgists manage to sustain a seemingly uninterrupted stream of air during their various activities?

The longest held, breath-induced and sustained musical note (last time I checked) was forty-seven minutes and six seconds. Impressive in the extreme!

The technique employed in this process is known as 'Circular Breathing,' although the good news is that – for relaxation purposes at least – you don't need to become anywhere near so proficient. In fact, it's more about slowing and steadying your breathing (thus avoiding a subconscious urge to hyperventilate during a panic attack), than expelling a continuous blast of air. The idea here is that during 'Circular Breathing,' you can't over-breathe. Hyperventilation occurs when the pace of your breathing eliminates more carbon dioxide than your body produces, leading to a variety of symptoms including dizziness and fainting.

The term 'Circular Breathing' derives its name from breathing in through the nose and out through the mouth. Lungs are filled to capacity nasally, then the air is blown out orally. As the lungs empty, the last bit of air is used to inflate the practitioner's cheeks. Squeezing those cheeks together to expel this final volume of air, another breath is taken through the nose.

The first difficulty a new student encounters is how to breathe in through the nose while squeezing out that last bit of air. For musicians, learning to alternate between the remaining air in their cheeks and the new air in their lungs without altering consistent pressure on the instrument, can be an issue. Thankfully we don't have to worry about any of that.

'Diaphragmatic Breathing' is a process of contracting the diaphragm, allowing your chest and belly to rise and expand. It is slow, deep breathing. When combined with the 'Circular Breathing' (in through the nose, out through the mouth) process above, this helps stabilize breathing, regulates oxygen intake, and interrupts the 'Fight or Flight' stress response. In other words: A brilliant way to short-circuit panic and fire up your body's in-built relaxation mechanism. It can also be used to combat insomnia, and as a general relaxation tool to reduce stress before it becomes problematic.

I suggest learning this exercise while laying down, or sitting comfortably if that is a problem. The process can certainly be used anywhere, but these postures make it easier to learn the technique and focus on your diaphragm.

Let's begin:

1. *Get comfortable on a bed or in a chair, allowing your limbs to go as loose as possible.*

2. *Place one hand on your chest and another in the area of your diaphragm (between tummy and breast bone is just fine).*

3. *Breathe slowly in through your nose, feeling your chest and tummy rise underneath your hands. Try counting slowly to five as you do this. It will help regulate the pace.*

4. *Hold your breath for another slow count of five. If this feels too uncomfortable at first, a couple of seconds will suffice.*

5. *Now release the air through your mouth to an additional slow count of five, letting your chest and tummy sink back down.*

6. *Once all air has been expelled, repeat steps 3 — 5 several more times until you feel the sensation of relaxation starting to manifest. It is important to go slow. If you can reduce the number of breaths taken to around five per minute while doing this, you will start to experience the benefits in no time. Ordinary breathing is in the 12 — 20 per minute range, while hyperventilation can be around three times that.*

7. *It is worth re-emphasizing the point about SLOWNESS above. When you conduct a deep-breathing exercise like this, your body receives around ten times the amount of oxygen than during shallow, chest breathing. If you do it quickly, the risk of hyperventilating rises exponentially, so PLEASE go slow. Because you are breathing with your abdomen, the extra air means your body is still receiving plenty of oxygen but at a calmer pace.*

Once you've got the hang of this, try it while standing up and without placing your hands on your body. Pretty soon, you will gain excellent control of your breathing at the drop of a hat. It's such a simple tool, which I have used in so many positive, life-enhancing ways and situations, they almost deserve their own book!

As mentioned in the chapter describing sleep difficulties, I came to find that a combination of Circular/Diaphragmatic Breathing and Progressive Muscular Relaxation was a dynamite combination for settling down into a good night's rest. To this day if my mind is swimming with busy thoughts and I can't get to sleep, I still use the same combination of tools I learned during those dark days of burnout.

When you first start doing this exercise, you may feel an urge to gulp air. It is important to resist this. When used during the first panic attack or two, the difference between an agitated rate of breathing close to hyperventilation and the ideal relaxed state this induces, can make you worry that your body isn't getting enough oxygen. Be assured it is, and keep that thought in the back of your mind. In fact, as previously mentioned, you are in fact taking in a lot more oxygen during abdominal breathing.

One positive side effect I and many others have found from making this a regular part of life, is that the body seems to start doing it subconsciously after a while. The sense of physical and emotional wellbeing that slow, circular, abdominal breathing induces pays many health and lifestyle dividends.

Panic attacks are another 'delightful,' unwanted common side effect of the burnout experience. They can strike at any time and their symptoms manifest suddenly with a combination of intense, unexplained fear (not necessarily related to any obvious situational stimuli) and typically four or more of the following additional symptoms:

- Dizziness, feeling faint or light-headed, unsteady on your feet, a sensation that you are falling or going to fall down
- Sweats (I found the base at the back of my neck was the most common spot)
- Shaking/trembling
- Heart palpitations and/or racing pulse
- Shortness of breath
- Hot/cold flushes, intense chills or heat sensations
- Numbness and tingling
- A sense of being detached from your body or feeling of unreality
- Choking and/or smothering sensations
- Fear of insanity (i.e. "I'm going mad!")
- Chest pains

- Abdominal discomfort/sudden nausea

- Sudden fear that you are dying or about to die

Thrilling stuff, hey?

What sets panic attacks apart from more generalised anxiety, is their sudden onset, intensity, and limited duration episodic nature. Most are over and done with in anything from five to twenty minutes. Due to the symptoms described above, it's not unusual to find people rushing to A&E convinced they are about to have a heart attack, or other life-threatening illness. The attacks can happen without warning, whether you feel anxious or calm. Sometimes their onset it brought on by stress triggers - like my encounter with the switched off computer - while at others there is no apparent cause.

To say that these nasty little internal assailants are both unpleasant and frightening, is quite an understatement. If you've already experienced at least one, you will have a fair idea what I'm talking about here. In fact, they are so frightening we can be tempted to make wholesale changes to our lifestyle and activities, to avoid anything that might induce one. This is unhelpful, and where the graded exposure techniques covered earlier in the book are a real boon. When I sat in a room with that computer for my allocated number of minutes each day, using NLP anchors and the breathing techniques here enabled me to fight off the effects of panic attacks caused by that stress trigger. Avoiding using a computer, being in a warm room, or driving a car for the rest of my life just wasn't practical.

Panic attacks are difficult and embarrassing to talk about. There is always that worry in the back of the mind that you are turning into a hypochondriac, or maybe going insane. As a general rule, those who are genuinely mad rarely worry about it or realise that they are, so you're probably not. The sudden onset of panic attacks (even during the absence of a notable stress trigger) can be quite frustrating. You might have had a really good week on the road to recovery, then BANG: three panic attacks strike out of the blue during the course of a single day. As with everything else, don't berate yourself if that happens. In fact, that's even pretty normal if it's any consolation to you. The nice thing about these breathing exercises is that they act as another helpful form of distraction. If you focus on the rise and fall, visualizing the breath moving in a circular motion in through your nose and out through your mouth, other thoughts are pushed aside (for a time at least). Sometimes this action of breaking a chain of negative thoughts, is just what you need to move forward.

The physical manifestation is a classic 'Fight or Flight' response by your body, but to an un-realistic, absent or invisible threat. We try to take in more oxygen with rapid over-breathing, adrenaline courses through our system, and muscles tense up ready to face whatever challenges may come.

As horrible as they are to endure, rest assured panic attacks are typically harmless.

That said, it is still worth a visit to a medical professional to rule out any underlying physical conditions. If the attack lasts longer than an hour after using these breathing exercises, your heartbeat seems irregular, or you experience ongoing chest pains or a sense of feeling unwell, I would strongly advise a trip to the doctor.

When I started driving again, the control I had learned from these techniques while working on my 'computer phobia' proved a real bonus. Panic attacks often occur in situations where an easy route of escape is not apparent. Cars, lifts/elevators, crowded shopping malls etc. are all typical places people experience them, even without an obviously stressful trigger or ingrained negative mental association present.

Graded exposure with the 'car phobia' commenced with me sitting in a stationary vehicle, starting and stopping the engine, then progressing to driving a short distance with a passenger who was also an experienced driver. This grew into driving solo and gradually longer journeys. All the while, 'Circular/Diaphragmatic Breathing' was used to fight off the onset of panic attacks and steady my pulse. If you can get it clear in your mind that (especially after getting a handle on your breathing) you are unlikely to pass out, you're not having a heart attack, and nothing really bad is going to happen; that also helps defuse the 'bomb.'

Panic attacks remind me of the frightened old man behind the screen in 'The Wizard of Oz,' who is pulling levers to project a scary face onto a large wall and seem more frightening than he is in reality. They're causing your bodily responses to lie to you about what is really going on, and filling your mind with outcomes that almost certainly won't happen. Don't believe a word of it, take charge of your breathing, and the villain will be shown for what he is in no time at all.

One of my longer initial journeys involved a forty-five minute drive to a large, indoor shopping mall one sunny weekday. I managed the car part of the outing with only minor worries, which didn't intensify thanks to the controlled breathing. NOTE: If you are not at the stage of being able to do the breathing without focussing your attention on it (it's nicer if you are in a situation/environment where you CAN allow yourself to focus on it, incidentally), DO NOT attempt this while driving. Please pull over to a safe and legal spot, conduct the exercise until you feel calm again, and then proceed on your journey when all is well and you can keep your concentration on the road where it belongs.

After I had been at the shopping mall for about half an hour, feeling generally okay, a sudden, full-blown panic attack with 'lights and sirens' jumped me out of nowhere. I had just emerged from an upstairs toilet, out into the large, glass-roofed atrium. While it was slightly warm and a little stuffy, there weren't that many people around and I hadn't felt uncomfortably hot. No worries or stress triggers were activated as far as I could tell. Next thing I knew, my neck was sweating, heart pounding, I felt hot, light-headed, dizzy, it seemed as though I was about to pass out and/or die, and I staggered to grab hold of a nearby railing. There was also a strong sense of falling (another reason for the rail grab). All around, the small number of folk nearby looked at me with expressions of curiosity. I think the way I held onto that railing for dear life, red-faced and panic-stricken probably got their attention. Maybe they thought I was on drugs or something? This is another case where you can start feeling embarrassed to go out. While I was somewhat pre-occupied with the attack to really care what anybody thought, once the peak intensity passed there came a strong sense of acting like some kind of social pariah. The attack might have lasted longer, had I not finally remembered all I had learned. I'd like to say I just switched into it effortlessly, but this was the first attack without an obvious trigger, and at the time I didn't know such things could occur. In my mind, I wondered if I was genuinely about to collapse and have another seizure as part of this mysterious burnout illness. Now I know better. Knowledge is a wonderful thing for driving out fear. Make it your ally, and you're halfway there.

I made a point of returning to that exact spot on a couple more journeys over the next few weeks. Sure enough, other attacks came. The first time I was ready, and jumped on it before the symptoms could really take hold. The next time, the panic attack barely made it out of the 'starting gate' before it was history. Defeating these things provides another welcome shot in the arm of confidence. A real boost.

As I write this, I am in the situation of having conquered my stress triggers many years ago as part of that initial recovery process. I've had another highly successful career in I.T, driven tens of thousands of miles alone by car, and enjoy a warm (if not overly stuffy) room. However, at certain periods on occasion throughout the last decade, I have experienced the odd panic attack without reason or warning. Sometimes this has been at the wheel of a vehicle, or even just lying in bed. I usually stop them in their tracks, and take the event as a signal to pause and closely examine what is going on in my life. Stress has a way of sneaking up on us, unnoticed. It's like the old story about a frog and boiling water. Put a live frog in a pan of boiling water, and it will jump right out. Sit the same frog in a pan of cool water and gradually turn up the heat, and it will sit there until it cooks. In that way panic attacks have become curious 'friends,' acting as barometers or doomsayers that the sky might fall if I don't pay attention.

While we're on the subject of bodily reactions, there's another simple tool you can use without learning anything: LAUGHTER. Now you might be thinking, *"Is this guy crazy? Right about now, laughing seems like the last thing I would want to do!"*

I completely understand, of course. However, many cultures and even modern medicine have identified the positive, health-giving, stress-busting effects of laughter on our human physiology. There's another old piece of Biblical wisdom in the seventeenth Proverb that sums it up in a nutshell, irrespective of one's personal belief system:

'A merry heart doeth good like a medicine: but a broken spirit drieth the bones.'

Or as Mark Twain put it:

'Against the assault of laughter, nothing can stand.'

I'd heard of this during my illness, but naturally I also didn't feel much like laughing, either. At home, we had some old comedy poetry records from years ago. They were simple, innocent humour about everyday things. In the evenings I'd put one on. Laughing didn't happen immediately or vigorously, but over time the cumulative effect with everything else added value and fuel to my upward trajectory.

A few years ago, some psychologists discovered that playing back recordings of people laughing could universally induce a positive emotional, psychological and physiological response without the need for an understood joke. Did you ever see/hear someone else laughing, and find yourself 'getting going' even though you had no idea what was so funny? Bingo!

Take a look at some of the popular video sharing sites on the Internet these days, and you'll discover compilations of human laughter that are quite uplifting. Sometimes these feature goofy home videos gone wrong, at others they may just be audio files of laughter itself. Simply type 'laughter' or 'contagious laughter' in the site's search box, then turn up the sound, click and enjoy. It's the simplest thing, even easier than learning slow, circular breathing from the abdomen. But sometimes the simplest things are the most effective. At a time when your mind and senses are typically overloaded, simple is REALLY GOOD.

CHAPTER 7 - THE WINDS OF CHANGE ARE BLOWING

HELPING TO INDUCE IDEAL PERFORMANCE OUTCOMES

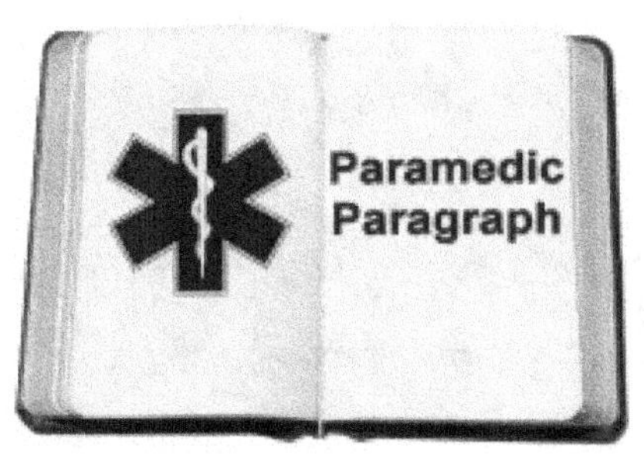

Positive Visualisation and Mental Rehearsal.

'Positive Visualisation' is about seeing a goal as accomplished, before it occurs in reality. A simple way to understand this idea is the old saying 'seeing is believing.'

'Mental Rehearsal' is imagined mental practice of performing a task or functioning in a specific situation, as opposed to actual practice. Its purpose is to hone and improve your confidence and performance when you do it for real.

I lump these two together in one technique, as the combination is a natural one that can dramatically change how you behave and react in certain situations (and consequently how others react to you). Think of 'Positive Visualisation' as the desired OUTCOME and 'Mental Rehearsal' as successfully completing the required PROCESS or STEPS along the way. When you do that, both their distinctiveness and complimentary natures should make a bit more sense.

Let's start with another simple exercise, then in the main text of the chapter I'll talk about how surprisingly common this practice is in everything from psychology to the world of business and professional sport.

1. *Choose a time when you can relax, uninterrupted. I tend to use this exercise at the start of a day before getting up, but any time that works for you is just fine.*

2. *Either lie down or sit comfortably, eyes closed.*

3. *Get a handle on your breathing and loosen any muscle tension. This is the perfect time to use the 'Progressive Muscular Relaxation' and 'Circular/Diaphragmatic Breathing' exercises we have already looked at. If you like, do those now then pick up this exercise from point number four below.*

4. *Visualize your goal as if it has already been completed successfully (for example: walking out of a potentially difficult meeting at work, after everything went really well).*

5. *Just like you did with setting NLP Anchors, clearly picture the scene, pump up the sounds and colours in your mind, and allow yourself to feel how relieved and happy you would be in that situation. As you fully embrace the feeling of it, there may be a tingling or whooshing sensation in your body that feels really good. If so, great! If not, don't worry and just keep seeing that successful outcome in your 'mind's eye.'*

6. *After allowing yourself to enjoy the experience of achieving your goal, imagine what you will see at the start of the activities required to get there (i.e. waiting outside the meeting room etc.). Try to picture this in the first person, rather than watching yourself like a spectator.*

7. *Now run through the various component parts on the road to your goal, imagining them going well. In the example of a meeting I have used thus far, see and hear yourself giving polite, professional responses that assert your own needs clearly. Feel the assurance of coming up with the correct words at just the right moment, and the other meeting participants reacting in a positive and engaged way to your input. How does that feel? Enjoy the sensation and know that all is well. Feel happy, competent and supported, whatever the particular goal or individual actions focus on.*

8. *Once you've run through the steps, it's sometimes worth playing them again. The reason is, later steps occasionally conjure up other positive possibilities for earlier ones. Plus, you are attempting to form a strong neural pathway in the brain, so a little repetition can be helpful anyway.*

9. *Finally, re-visualize the successful goal outcome and feel it again. Open your eyes, smile, and congratulate yourself with comforting words of positive reinforcement on a job well done.*

The primary purpose here is to reduce stress and anxiety, boost confidence, and help yourself perform naturally at your best, without interference from negative, subconscious internal dialogues.

If this is a new concept to you, there might be some concerns about being sucked into the *'you can have anything you imagine'* type mantra of popular self-help gurus that I alluded to earlier. Now, it's not my place to rubbish the views or beliefs of others, but that's not what this is really all about. I could imagine myself winning an Olympic gold medal and feel really great about it. Does that mean if I partook in an Olympic sport (without training hard and putting-in years of practice), it would actually happen? Of course not! Action is required. Just because you picture something going well, does that mean you are definitely creating such an outcome? Well, there are some Quantum Physicists who might say that at an 'energetic' level, we are influencing the result to a degree. Maybe years from now there will be hard science brought into the mainstream to back up such a concept, and I certainly don't want to 'poo poo' it. However, I'm not peddling that concept per-se. What science certainly DOES know about this practice, is that (especially in relation to physical actions and movement) when we visualize imagery, our brain neurons interpret it as real-life action. These impulses initiate a new cluster of brain cells dedicated to creating memories and learned behaviour, known as a 'Neural Pathway.' The result primes our system to behave in certain ways consistent with that imagery, even without physically conducting the activity to create a 'memory' in real life.

This is one reason professional sportspeople understand and

use this technique on a regular basis. An athlete competing in a hurdle race or high jump 'sees' themselves successfully achieving their activity. Then they mentally run through every part of the race/event, pushing forwards, breaking imaginary barriers and being their absolute best to get 'in the zone.' Combined with all the actual hard work and training, it really helps them produce positive results. Worries and distractions about the event that could affect their performance are cast aside. Their brains experience the effect of successfully completing the activity, as if they had just done it for real. This in turn strengthens that neural pathway. Does all that mean they will definitely win the event? If it did, every race full of athletes practising such techniques would obviously be a draw. Clearly it isn't, but the practice certainly helps them compete at an optimum level.

The benefits of 'Positive Visualisation' and 'Mental Rehearsal' are not only limited to sport and intensive physical activity, however. From parents and romantic partners contemplating difficult interventions with children/partners, through business people delivering presentations, undertaking job interviews and seeking to improve their communication and/or performance, to psychologists working with patients trying to overcome phobias, low self-esteem and confidence problems, this same basic principle is another helpful tool in the toolbox of life. Essentially it's a way to supplement actual practice with imagined practice. Actual practice that always or regularly goes wrong is not entirely helpful. By adding a form of practice where everything always goes right (remembering that your system can't properly distinguish between a real event and a vividly imagined one in many ways) can provide a confidence boost leading to actual, better real-world practice outcomes in the future.

None of this is of course a guarantee of success, or that the genuine situation will play out as imagined. I can sit here until I'm a hundred years old, imagining and feeling how great it would be if the sky rained chocolate drops. I'll get a good deal older and not eat any chocolate along the way.

As previously mentioned, I'm not into belittling the beliefs of others. In my varied and interesting life, I have experienced a plethora of such ideas. On numerous occasions for myself and others, I have witnessed the power of 'faith' in an outcome appear to produce amazing results. Sometimes this was clearly because the holder of such faith then used it to focus on inspired activity that brought about their goal. At others, there didn't seem to be any particular correlation between activity (or lack thereof) and the result. The universe is a curious and wonderful place, I think.

However, the purpose of this book is to provide tools ANYBODY can use, without the need to subscribe to a particular philosophy.

What I can definitely say from the many times I have used this technique successfully, is that (at times of stress especially) it lightens the mental and emotional load and makes intimidating situations a lot less scary. Seemingly impossible barriers have become effortless, toothless tigers to defeat. After visualizing a successful outcome and mentally rehearsing its steps, I have typically enjoyed natural, unhindered performance 'on the day.' For that reason alone, it's worth giving it a fair hearing.

Let's look at a pivotal day during my recovery, where this certainly came in handy.

I'd formally resigned from the job as 'Senior Technical Analyst.' HR placed me 'At Risk,' which was a status with a limited time window allowing staff to find another post working for the organisation, rather than face immediate termination. My own time was running out. During the various secondments I tried, one was back in the IT Training department, which proved a perfect fit for me. Unfortunately, there had been no actual vacancies available.

Suddenly, a temporary one-year contract appeared to train a specific new branch of staff in various IT systems. If I got it, this at least gave me twelve months of guaranteed work at a level commensurate with my skills and qualifications. In other words, I would achieve my goal of returning to life as a properly productive member of the organisation, even if that meant facing unemployment once it was over. I put in the paperwork and was offered an interview, during which I needed to deliver a training presentation on a business-related IT subject. This of course involved a decent amount of computer time while putting together a quality product.

However, since resigning from the software development role, I had unsurprisingly made excellent progress in fully destroying the computing stress trigger. Without the prospect of returning to that old job hanging over me like the proverbial 'Sword of Damocles,' things had become considerably easier.

Presentation ready to go, I knew there were other potential candidates in the offing whose performance that day I would need to surpass. Only one vacancy was on offer. If I didn't get it, I'd be on the unemployment line within a couple of months. These were intimidating thoughts.

During burnout and our recovery from it, 'all or nothing thinking' and 'Catastrophizing' are common mental responses to stressful situations. That is to say, we tend to focus on one of two possible outcomes to any given situation - either really good or really bad – and are unable to consider the many (often positive) nuanced alternatives and middle ground options. Or, we think that not only is everything going to go wrong, it's going to go SPECTACULARLY wrong. Neither of these responses is helpful or realistic, and they can develop into new patterns of learned behaviour if left unchecked.

I weighed out the positives and negatives in a rational manner, with a simple and common set of questions such as:

1. What is the issue?
2. What's the worst that could happen?
3. How would I manage if that happened?

4. What is a more positive way to view this issue?

This is a helpful way of succinctly distilling a problem down on paper, when your mind is clouded or racing with various worries and negative outcomes in a seemingly uncontrollable fashion.

For the upcoming presentation and interview, my piece of paper read similar to the following:

1. What is the issue?

If I don't get this post, I will most likely find myself without a job and income, facing the prospect of trying to secure a new career. This will involve interviews with the dreaded question: *'So why did you leave your last employer?'* and subsequent possible negative bias from my truthful answer to it, making further employment opportunities impossible. (Notice 'all or nothing thinking' and 'Catastrophizing' in full swing here).

2. What's the worst that could happen?

I would have to find another job/means of generating an income.

3. How would I manage if that happened?

I've conducted a number of different careers, so would attempt something new. During interview, I could easily explain that I suffered from a toxic work environment and am now healthy, well and looking to move in a different employment direction.

4.   What is a more productive way to view this issue?

Burnout and work-stress related illness is a modern, well-documented epidemic across all strata of society, rather than a bizarre neurosis affecting a handful of 'losers.'   Reasonably intelligent employers will know and understand this, also being aware of the many thousands of people currently switching careers for similar reasons. During such an interview, if the topic even came up in a big way, I could wax lyrical about my fantastic and self-disciplined recovery. I might tell the positive story of my journey back to productive employment. One that ultimately only ended because no current vacancies were available, and I had sensibly resigned from the job that caused the problems in the first place. It's the tale of a take-charge, positive, committed worker (also the view of HR) that anyone with an ounce of sense would be happy to employ.

As you can probably imagine, just getting this down on paper already made me feel a lot better about the issue. Especially after I had written and re-read the final question and answer a few times. Suddenly my approaching 'high jump' didn't seem quite so high, and the prospect of failing to clear it no longer felt like the end of the world.

In the run up to interview day, I used 'Positive Visualisation' and 'Mental Rehearsal' to get myself relaxed and in the flow of how I wanted the event to pan out. All the while I now realised that whatever happened, everything really would be okay one way or another.

Walking away from a stellar presentation and Q & A session where I could hardly believe the inspired responses coming out of my own mouth, I felt happier and more at peace than even my earlier imaginings had allowed. I got the job and started working there a few days later.

Over the coming years I would have to undergo this almost identical process several more times, for a variety of one year contracts with the same unit. Each time I had to deliver a new presentation, undergo an interview, and deal with eager candidate competition for the post in question. Each time I used these same processes to help me perform at my best, and (thankfully) secure an additional year of work.

Finally, a permanent member of staff in the department moved on, and I got to compete for that job too. It was a role I held very successfully until the end of 2013. But, more on that as we wrap all of this up in the next chapter, and consider our individual futures together…

CHAPTER 8 – WHEREVER THE ROAD MAY LEAD

THE ONWARD JOURNEY

"I can't believe I actually get paid for doing this!" It was a phrase I uttered to myself on a number of very happy occasions over the next eight years. There can be few aspects of life more rewarding, than finding yourself in an employment situation that elicits such a response. Sadly, it's an all too uncommon turn of phrase, and - as I eventually discovered - only a few minor changes in the work, environment and staffing (those three big stressors) around you can drastically alter this perception and its impact on your wellbeing.

My work as an IT Trainer was paying massive dividends for the organisation, the general public we served, the reputation of our unit and my subsequent individual happiness and job satisfaction. I lost four Stone in weight in under two months prior to commencing the post, then took up a new hobby as a modern jive dancer and occasional voluntary dance coach to improve and maintain my physical fitness levels. A keen walker, I've never been a particularly sporty person. If your life - especially your work life - is quite sedentary, I highly recommend finding some form of regular physical activity as a way to boost health and energy. This procures the added benefit of simultaneously releasing feel-good endorphins that reduce and combat the effects of stress on your system. It will make a big difference to your resilience in the face of life's challenges, along with potentially increasing your longevity and warding off common diseases. This doesn't have to be a competitive team sport or unduly strenuous activity, if that's not your thing. Find something you will enjoy and look forward to doing, then it won't become a laborious chore or effort.

Over the next few years, I got to offer support and advice to a number of colleagues, acquaintances and friends suffering the effects of burnout. Many of them received instruction in the streamlined techniques found in this book, which worked so well for me. It was the positive effect of these interventions that led those people to encourage me in creating this compact help guide. While I was never formally a counsellor, the office I eventually shared with one other colleague became known as a sanctuary or 'safe haven' when work and personal storms hit. I had a comfortable chair in the corner which folk loved to sit in and unload, followed by enjoying a few chocolate counters from the pot on my desk. As time wore on and our organisation suffered significant restructuring and financial cutbacks, the chair rarely seemed to grow cold.

I've already described some types of people I really can't stand. We had one such individual on the team, who had inherited a supervisory post by default that she was neither qualified nor fit to hold. Not being one to suffer fools gladly, I tolerated her professionally as much as possible, without putting up with any of her nonsense if it directly interfered with my own work. If I had a Pound for every time someone landed in my comfy chair after suffering at the hands of her lies, game playing and being required to pick-up her workload, I might have contemplated early retirement. Regrettably, the overall unit manager lacked the backbone to confront her, and so none of her abuses ever found their way onto the woman's falsely spotless employment record.

Around 2011, a number of wholesale changes began to degrade our professional performance and personal contentment with the job. Firstly, the IT and Training arms of our organisation were unified with those of another, who worked in very different ways. Suddenly staff were required to travel long distances to what was essentially a different 'firm' and deliver courses for them. Then amidst budget cutbacks, all trainers were suddenly expected to 'Income Generate.' That is to say, we had to take the formidable reputation our excellent work had earned, and use it to sell training to external agencies. This involved considerable logistical nightmares, extensive travel, bureaucratic headaches and functioning in a 'sales' capacity we never signed up to. The 'Income Generation' function was now re-written into our 'Job Description,' as if it had been part of the employment contract. Our reward for doing this? Absolutely nothing! After one such engagement that placed an unnecessarily negative burden on my health, I decided to ignore any further such requests. On paper, I was available to sell my well-known and sought-after courses to the masses. In reality, I quietly turned down every opportunity presented, stating that we were unavailable. Since my own 'proper' workload (i.e. the job I had been employed to do at interview) was still there and ever increasing, this was no falsehood. External training just wasn't worth it, other than to those who reaped the benefit of my labour. Those beneficiaries were neither me, nor even our team and its budget.

As if that hadn't been enough, training staff were then pressured to halve the duration of courses and consider simple student attendance rather than actual trainer assessment as a 'pass.' I didn't study at night school to get my teaching qualifications, so I could betray everything that stood for. Many others clearly felt the same. In no time at all, our hard-won reputation for excellence would disappear into the gutter. Nobody with an ounce of integrity or professional pride was going to tolerate the situation very much longer, and those who could afford it, slowly began to quit.

In the early spring of 2013, I was driving home on a particularly sunny afternoon. Despite the previously detailed challenges and annoyances surrounding my work, I was still heavily engaged in a ground-breaking project that I absolutely loved. Many was the time on a Friday night that I'd still be working three hours after everyone else had gone home, because I was so happily invested in the job at hand. This in itself speaks volumes on how we feel about our work, affecting the personal resources we have to cope with it. Even so, too much of a 'good thing' can still have a negative impact on your system. I think it did on mine, to an extent.

From out of nowhere, a full-blown panic attack struck me at the wheel. Deciding to play it safe, I pulled over to an appropriate spot and conducted some 'Circular/Diaphragmatic Breathing' exercises until the manifestations subsided. The whole episode emerged out of left field as a complete and utter surprise. In fact, I couldn't even remember the last time I had suffered an attack like that. Quickly, I began to run down a list of stressful encounters over the last few months. There had been a situation with a romantic ex-partner, who spitefully attempted to create career trouble for me. Several nights were spent sitting up in A&E with my dear old Dad, as he suffered various post-surgery complications. Then of course, there were the assorted other little contributors I've already written about. Despite feeling generally pretty happy, the cumulative health impact had obviously been greater than I fully realised. Either that, or I just pushed it all down and hadn't been paying attention. Thanks for the wake-up call, panic attack!

The next couple of days at the office would be dedicated to admin, rather than classroom training. So, I phoned my supervisor (somebody I had also helped recover from burnout), told her what occurred, booked two days leave, and disappeared to a county I liked to go walking in. By the following Monday I had sorted myself out for work, and carried on as usual without any further negative side-effects. I knew what to do, employed the various techniques detailed in this book, reflected on and positively re-framed how I felt about any residual stresses from the difficult times, and made a plan to reduce some of my excess working hours for the foreseeable future. All that did the job nicely.

That summer, I attended an external conference organised by a software company whose products I used in one of my subject specialisms. For many years I had found new and creative ways for our staff to enhance their job performance, with innovative uses of the software. This had been translated into complimentary training courses, support material, and new working practices. In front of a massive assembled audience, representing many professional spheres, the company called me up on stage to deliver an award recognising my achievements. A banner day in any career, and no mistake. Along with this, my revised professional trajectory had also garnered a national award for the team, two personal internal awards for myself, and a medal from the British Prime Minister. You could say that I considered the recovery goal I initially set in 2004, to have been well and truly hit.

"John, you'd better come upstairs. I've something to tell you that you're not going to like." The face of my normally-jolly and much-cherished female supervisor, Diane, evidenced grave concern. It was September, 2013. I assembled in the office with two other colleagues

who reported to the same lady. It transpired that the joint 'firm' we had effectively become, was working on a bespoke software project written by a company who were the 'lowest bidder' in every negative connotation of the term. The massive training implications for this had been handed to the team supervisor I previously mentioned in a distasteful light. Several staff from both organisations already either quit or refused to work with her, and she had been relieved of the responsibility. Instead, people at the other place (who didn't know our team), decided that my supervisor would assume the project role and her staff would now instead be managed by the walking nightmare. Diane looked at me. *'I told them if they do this, John will resign.'* She knew me well and wasn't wrong. This was now a matter of principle and somebody had to finally take a stand.

Helpfully, the following week I'd booked a break to replace a holiday cut short earlier in the year. While this proved anything but restful due to the choices I was now forced to consider, it at least allowed me to get properly quiet and decide which course of action to take. I reflected on the increasing negative requirements placed on our unit, the unprofessional demands to deliver training 'in name only,' plus the constant rumblings that massive redundancies might not be far away. Then I realistically visualised life reporting to the useless woman, and the constant fight against lies and games that would demand of me on an almost daily basis. This was based on the real-world experiences of so many others I had consoled during their times of trouble with her. The red line was clear: I might be willing to carry on working there for now while considering the future, but not with that woman as my supervisor. I wrote a letter to senior management, clearly stating my position. This politely informed them that I now considered this both a personal health and integrity issue, but was willing to discuss supervision by any other staff member they chose. Four other managers had gladly offered to take my low-impact, self-managing person on board.

Since the woman had never been formally reprimanded for her abuse, it came as quite a surprise to HR when they discovered various staff members had been individually collating evidence against her for some years. This was now assembled into a book by a designated investigator, amounting to several hundred pages. I've said it before and I'll say it again: People are the biggest stressors.

Senior management informed me that they were working to resolve the situation, but that I had to report to the woman for now. I'd heard this sort of thing before. So, I tendered my resignation with a heavy heart and little idea what to do next. After fifteen years of service and with my career on a high, it was the right time. A wonderful position had decayed into something intolerable. All good things…

I have no idea whether this decision influenced the eventual outcome, but the next day with my other colleagues now refusing to work for the woman and facing possible disciplinary action, the troublemaker was given a golden handshake to leave. All the remaining staff talent - not on the cusp of retirement - either transferred to other units or followed me out the door within a year.

It came as no surprise. Carrying on there was no longer a realistic option for anyone with genuine value. The only thing sadder than people who give up and leave, are people who give up and stay.

Over the next few years I returned twice. The first time was after being invited to receive yet another award 'posthumously.' That busy final project I had been so engaged with (an interactive video e-learning series for the whole organisation) proved so phenomenally successful, other firms were lining up to try and buy it. The award recognised my achievement. The second time I returned, was as an independent consultant to deliver a bespoke training day for some of their analytical staff. This enabled me to see how far the organisation had degraded, with budgets squeezed so tight the classroom corridor water coolers had even been removed!

On hearing about my departure, the outpouring of positive staff communications I had received was not only touching, but also served to illustrate an important point: My training career had made a GENUINE impact of the work success and happiness of our people. In a situation where measuring training success had now become *if you bother to turn up, you've passed,'* this was especially good to hear. Along with the comment I quoted earlier in the book, here are a sample of just three that illustrate this. The last offers simple, sage advice on self-care in the light of career choices. In fact, I was quite taken aback by how many people wrote and said they had previously or were now experiencing work-stress related issues.

'I would like to personally thank you for all the help, support and knowledge that you have supplied me with during the short time that I have been within the Analyst team. Your genuine enthusiasm, endless knowledge and ability to pass this on to others is something I aspire to.'

'Ohhhh John, we are all distraught here. That is such sad and upsetting news, many in the office opened your e-mail at the same time and I walked into a room full of 'nooooo!!' or 'AHHHHHHHH!!' to find out that you were leaving.'

'I have nothing but the utmost respect for you and know you are too good for the role you are performing. Life is so short that you need to make the most of the talents you have in a way which enriches yourself as well as others.'

This whole situation caused some of those classic burnout symptoms to rear their ugly heads. Chest pains, sweats, shaking, over-breathing etc. all let me know I needed to sort myself out. Yet again, it had been a steady build-up now starting to make itself known. I left the job in late October, and decided upon a complete rest from work until January.

During this time I started a regular walking blog, using my geographic skills to post routes online for people to enjoy, including aspects of local history. On one of those walks, I encountered the familiar face of a man strolling the opposite way with his wife. Sure enough, it was the doctor who had been of little use during my burnout. The man who thought there was nothing wrong with me. We got chatting, and I discovered he had also eventually suffered burnout and a breakdown just like myself, while his wife nursed him back to health. Now resigned from the medical profession, he went on regular walks to maintain his wellbeing. This didn't make me gloat at all. I felt sorry for him, and shared my own story since our last encounter. As we parted, his wife told me not to overdo whatever I chose to work on next. It was an affirming experience, adding a strong sense of closure to those initial days of my illness nearly a decade before.

In January 2014, I commenced studying for further qualifications - soon attained. I developed my subject specialism into a new set of courses that were solely my own intellectual property. These were delivered as training services direct to a number of organisations, until their own financial cutbacks made that no longer viable. Another former colleague - who had resigned in protest over mounting professional concerns - circulated my CV at a university, and I soon became a sessional lecturer on two of their campuses. In addition, I also edited a book for a client in Switzerland and (perhaps proudest achievement of all) wrote a number of small computer applications for a Spanish company. I had vowed never to go back to software development, and as a long term option wouldn't even consider it. All of those mini programming projects were less than a week long. At the end of each week, my mind was racing, neck aching. Clearly, the correct overall career decision had been made. But, actually being able to write software again without suffering panic attacks, enabled me to fully realise that I had conquered my enemy. It was a pretty great feeling, I can tell you!

As I write this, my professional life is in another state of uncertain flux. Indeed, it's the only reason I've finally found time to sit down and tell my story. What I do know, is that everything I learned on that difficult journey is still relevant today. Wherever the road may lead, that knowledge and these tools will help me make good career choices and survive the sometimes mental world of the modern workplace or other life challenges.

So, how about you?

Because my own burnout experience centred on work/life balance issues, those have been the overriding focus of this book. Also, because work is such a big part of our lives, this is a fairly typical cause. However, burnout can happen as a result of stress in a number of situations, such as bereavement or even buying and moving into a new home. It's not always a single nor professionally-related stressor or event that takes us over the edge, and we might very much look forward to being back at a job we enjoy.

My hope for you, is that by considering the story I have laid bare and using the helpful, natural exercises and techniques included herein; you will regain your health, work out what went wrong, and find the wisdom and courage to make any necessary life changes however great or small.

I said at the start that this was neither an extensive nor scholarly treatise on the topic of burnout. That was never my intention. But, if it has proven a companion on that long, dark road to recovery, offered some solidarity, comfort and given you tools to help, then I have succeeded in what I set out to achieve. Hopefully there has been just enough information and content to start you off, without filling and burdening your mind with unnecessary details.

During the first year of my recovery, I read a lot about the 'Slow Movement.' This covers the entire gamut from 'Slow Food' to 'Slow Sex' and everything in between. In an ever-connected and always-on world that moves way faster than our physiology was designed to assimilate, it's good to make a conscious effort to slow down, observe and enjoy. But it is a continual practise. Have you ever gone from the country to the city on a train? When you stepped off at your destination, I'm willing to bet you suddenly found yourself rushing, because everyone around you started rushing. Did you really need to rush? Was the minute or so you might have actually saved that important you'd rather arrive with your gut in a knot, mind racing, and shoulders tense? Probably not.

This morning I went for a regular constitutional walk around my country market town. As I approached a churchyard, the cherry blossom was making the most of a blue and sunny sky. Truly beautiful. Then I paused from rushing past - my mind previously filled with this book - and forced myself to actually STOP. It took several goes until I was no longer pushing to break away. In that moment, I allowed all my senses to register their surroundings, slowed my breathing and took in and fully enjoyed that free, gorgeous vista. The increased sense of relaxation and personal wellbeing this initiated was palpable. Then, the opening words of W. H. Davies' classic poem 'Leisure' were suddenly called to mind:

What is this life if, full of care,

We have no time to stand and stare.'

Don't let anybody belittle you for suffering this condition. Burnout is an experience shared by a large number of people, representing some of the best and brightest talent and intellect the human race has to offer. Rest assured, you are in VERY good company.

May good health and happiness be yours, now and always.